CROHN'S DISEASE DIET COOKBOOK FOR BEGINNERS

NATALIE BROWN

TABLE OF CONTENTS

WHAT IS CROHN'S DISEASE?

Crohn's disease is a type of inflammatory bowel disease (IBD). It causes inflammation of your digestive tract, which can lead to abdominal pain, severe diarrhea, fatigue, weight loss and malnutrition.

Inflammation caused by Crohn's disease can involve different areas of the digestive tract in different people. This inflammation often spreads into the deeper layers of the bowel.

Crohn's disease can be both painful and debilitating, and sometimes may lead to life-threatening complications.

While there's no known cure for Crohn's disease, therapies can greatly reduce its signs and symptoms and even bring about long-term remission and healing of inflammation. With treatment, many people with Crohn's disease are able to function well.

SYMPTOMS

When the disease is active, signs and symptoms may include:

- Diarrhea
- Fever
- Fatigue
- Abdominal pain and cramping
- Blood in your stool
- Mouth sores
- Reduced appetite and weight loss
- Pain or drainage near or around the anus due to inflammation from a tunnel into the skin (fistula)
- Other signs and symptoms
- People with severe Crohn's disease may also experience:
- Inflammation of skin, eyes and joints
- Inflammation of the liver or bile ducts
- Kidney stones
- Iron deficiency (anemia)

- Delayed growth or sexual development, in children

CAUSES

- **Immune system.** It's possible that a virus or bacterium may trigger Crohn's disease; however, scientists have yet to identify such a trigger. When your immune system tries to fight off the invading microorganism, an abnormal immune response causes the immune system to attack the cells in the digestive tract, too.
- **Heredity.** Crohn's is more common in people who have family members with the disease, so genes may play a role in making people more susceptible. However, most people with Crohn's disease don't have a family history of the disease.

RISK FACTORS

- **AGE.** Crohn's disease can occur at any age, but you're likely to develop the condition when you're young. Most people who develop Crohn's disease are diagnosed before they're around 30 years old.
- **ETHNICITY.** Although Crohn's disease can affect any ethnic group, whites have the highest risk, especially people of Eastern European (Ashkenazi) Jewish descent. However, the incidence of Crohn's disease is increasing among Black people who live in North America and the United Kingdom.
- **FAMILY HISTORY.** You're at higher risk if you have a first-degree relative, such as a parent, sibling or child, with the disease. As many as 1 in 5 people with Crohn's disease has a family member with the disease.
- **CIGARETTE SMOKING.** Cigarette smoking is the most important controllable risk factor for developing Crohn's disease. Smoking also leads to more-severe disease

and a greater risk of having surgery. If you smoke, it's important to stop.

WHAT SHOULD I EAT?

It's not always easy knowing what foods best fuel your body, especially when you have Crohn's disease or ulcerative colitis. Your diet and nutrition are a major part of life with inflammatory bowel disease (IBD), yet there is no single diet that works for everyone.

Nutrition affects not just your IBD symptoms, but also your overall health and well-being. Without proper nutrients, the symptoms of your Crohn's disease or ulcerative colitis can cause serious complications, including nutrient deficiencies, weight loss, and malnutrition.

We have several tips for a healthy diet that's well-balanced and nutrient rich. These tips are for educational purposes only. You should work with your doctor or a dietitian specializing in IBD to help you develop a personalized meal plan.

Watch our Facebook Live conversation with Emily Haller, registered dietitian at Michigan Medicine! Tune in to hear Emily review diet facts, debunk myths, speak about restrictions, and highlight ongoing research.

FOOD PREPARATION AND MEAL PLANNING

While there is no one-size-fits-all for meal planning, these tips can help guide you toward better daily nutrition:

- Eat four to six small meals daily.
- Stay hydrated — drink enough to keep your urine light yellow to clear — with water, broth, tomato juice, or a rehydration solution.
- Drink slowly and avoid using a straw, which can cause you to ingest air, which may cause gas.

- Prepare meals in advance, and keep your kitchen stocked with foods that you tolerate well (see list below).
- Use simple cooking techniques — boil, grill, steam, poach.
- Use a food journal to keep track of what you eat and any symptoms you may experience.

EATING WHEN YOU ARE IN A FLARE

There are certain foods you may want to avoid when you are in an IBD flare, and others that may help you get the right amount of nutrients, vitamins, and minerals without making your symptoms worse.

Your healthcare team may put you on an elimination diet, in which you avoid certain foods in order to identify which trigger symptoms. This process will help you identify common foods to avoid during a flare. Elimination diets should only be done under the supervision of your healthcare team and a dietitian so they can make sure you are still receiving the necessary nutrients.

Some foods may trigger cramping, bloating, and/or diarrhea. Many trigger foods should also be avoided if you have been diagnosed with a stricture, a narrowing of the intestine caused by inflammation or scar tissue, or have had a recent surgery. Certain foods can be easier to digest and can provide you with the necessary nutrients your body needs.

FOOD TO AVOID

- Lactose: sugar found in dairy, such as milk, cream cheese, and soft cheeses Lean protein: fish, lean cuts of pork, white meat poultry, soy, eggs, and firm tofu
- Non-absorbable sugars: sorbitol, mannitol, and other sugar alcohols found in sugar-free gum, candy, ice cream, and certain types of fruits and juices such as pear, peach, and prune Refined grains: sourdough, potato or

gluten-free bread, white pasta, white rice, and oatmeal

- Sugary foods: pastries, candy, and juices Fully cooked, seedless, skinless, non-cruciferous vegetables: asparagus tips, cucumbers, potatoes, and squash
- High fat foods: butter, coconut, margarine, and cream, as well as fatty, fried, or greasy food Oral nutritional supplements or homemade protein shakes: ask your doctor or your dietitian about what supplements may fit your nutritional needs
- Alcohol and caffeinated drinks: beer, wine, liquor, soda, and coffee
- Spicy foods: "hot" spices

CROHN'S DISEASE DIET RECIPES

BANANA OVERNIGHT OATS

INGREDIENTS

- 1 cup old-fashioned rolled oats
- 1 cup milk of choice (like oat milk)
- 2 teaspoons pure maple syrup
- 1 teaspoon vanilla extract
- 1 banana, sliced
- 1 tablespoon natural peanut butter (or nut butter of choice)

INSTRUCTIONS

1. Combine oats, milk, maple syrup, and vanilla in a small bowl and whisk together.
2. Divide mixture evenly between two mason jars.
3. Top each jar with sliced banana and drizzle peanut butter over the top.

4. Refrigerate for 4 or more hours. Enjoy hot or cold.

AVOCADO TOAST TOPPED WITH SCRAMBLED EGGS

INGREDIENTS

- 2 eggs
- 1/2 ripe avocado
- Pinch of salt and black pepper
- 1/2 tablespoon fresh lemon juice
- 2 slices sourdough or gluten-free bread, toasted

INSTRUCTIONS

1. Grease a frying pan with a bit of olive oil or cooking spray. When it's hot, scramble eggs for 1–2 minutes, or until fully cooked. (For an easier and more even scramble, you can crack the eggs into a bowl, mix them, and then pour them into the pan when it's hot.)
2. Mash avocado in a small bowl. Add salt and pepper, then add lemon juice and mix with a fork or spoon.

3. Divide avocado mash between toast slices and spread evenly.
4. Top toast with scrambled eggs.

STRAWBERRY, CUCUMBER, AND FETA SALAD

INGREDIENTS

- 1 cup sliced fresh strawberries
- 1 cup sliced cucumber
- 2 tablespoons crumbled feta cheese
- 1/2 tablespoon olive oil
- 1/2 tablespoon apple cider vinegar
- 1 grilled chicken breast (suggested)

INSTRUCTIONS

1. Add strawberries and cucumber to a salad bowl.
2. Top with feta.
3. Drizzle oil and vinegar over salad and toss gently.
4. Slice chicken breast, if using, and add to top of salad.

MEAT AND VEGETABLE ROLL-UPS

INGREDIENTS

- low FODMAP vegetables (such as cucumbers, celery, carrots, or bell peppers)
- deli-sliced ham or turkey breast

INSTRUCTIONS

1. Slice vegetables into matchsticks or small pieces.
2. Place a handful of vegetable slices onto 1–2 slices of deli meat, then roll into a burrito shape.
3. You can add toothpicks to hold the rolls together or eat them as they are.

BAKED LEMON CHICKEN AND SWEET POTATOES

INGREDIENTS

- 3 large sweet potatoes
- 1 cup low sodium chicken broth
- 1/2 cup fresh lemon juice (from 2 large lemons)

- 1/4 cup olive oil
- 1 teaspoon ground turmeric
- 1 teaspoon dried oregano
- 1/2 teaspoon salt
- 1/2 teaspoon pepper
- 3 boneless, skinless chicken breasts

INSTRUCTIONS

1. Preheat oven to 400°F (200°C).
2. Peel sweet potatoes to reduce their fiber content, if you'd like. Cut sweet potatoes into cubes.
3. Combine broth, lemon juice, oil, turmeric, oregano, salt, and pepper in a mixing bowl and whisk together.
4. Arrange sweet potatoes in a 9 x 13 baking pan. Place chicken breasts over sweet potatoes. Pour lemon mixture over chicken and sweet potatoes.
5. Roast in oven for 1 hour.

CRISPY BAKED PEANUT TOFU

INGREDIENTS

- 12 ounces extra-firm tofu
- 3 tablespoons coconut aminos
- 3 tablespoons water
- 2 tablespoons natural peanut butter (or nut butter of choice)
- 2 tablespoons pure maple syrup
- 1 tablespoon grated fresh ginger
- 1 zucchini

INSTRUCTIONS

1. Press tofu to get rid of water (you can do this by wrapping it in paper towels and placing a heavy bowl or pan on top of it for about 30 minutes). Cut tofu into 1-inch cubes.
2. Combine coconut aminos, water, peanut butter, maple syrup, and ginger in a mixing bowl and whisk together.
3. Pour mixture over tofu cubes. Cover and refrigerate for 1 hour.
4. Preheat oven to 400°F (200°C).

5. Slice zucchini.

6. Spread marinated tofu and sliced zucchini on a sheet pan. Spray with cooking spray for extra crispiness.

7. Bake for 30 minutes, or until tofu and zucchini are crispy around edges.

MISO RAMEN SOUP

INGREDIENTS

- ½ cup miso white or yellow
- 4 cups water
- 4 cups vegetable broth
- 2 tablespoons seaweed nori or wakame, soaked in water for two minutes, drained & rinsed
- 2 cups chopped greens chard, kale, or spinach
- 1 cup cubed firm or extra firm tofu about half a 15-oz package
- 2 cakes of ramen noodles 4 servings, if you are substituting another noodle
- 1 cup chopped green onion

INSTRUCTIONS

1. Whisk the miso into one cup of the water until it is smooth with no clumps. Set aside.
2. Bring the broth and remaining 3 cups water to a simmer.
3. Add the seaweed, greens, tofu, and ramen, and simmer for 5 to 7 minutes.
4. Remove from heat and stir in the miso.
5. Serve in a big bowl with green onion sprinkled generously on top.

EASY AIP GUACAMOLE

INGREDIENTS

- 5 avocados
- 2 minced shallots
- 1 tsp garlic powder
- 1 1/2 tsp sea salt
- Juice of 1 1/2 limes
- Optional: chopped cilantro or parsley, lime wedges to garnish

INSTRUCTIONS

1. Add the avocado (de-skinned and de-pitted) to the bowl with the rest of the ingredients. Mix really well to the consistency you like. A potato masher is helpful here! Serve with a variety of foods to dip in.

DAIRY-FREE MASHED POTATOES

INGREDIENTS

- 2 pounds potatoes (peeled, chopped into cubes)
- 1 teaspoon salt
- ½ cup light stock or bone broth
- ¼ cup olive oil
- 1-2 cloves garlic (minced)
- 1 tablespoon fresh rosemary (finely chopped)
- 1 teaspoon fresh cracked black pepper
- ½ teaspoon salt

INSTRUCTIONS

2. Add potatoes and salt to pot of boiling water, making sure water covers top of potatoes. Boil until you can easily pierce potatoes with fork.
3. Strain potatoes, return to pot, place back on stove (with heat turned off).
4. Add oil, stock, and garlic, mashing with potato masher until desired creaminess. Or, place all ingredients into a food processor until just blended together (being careful not to over blend or it can become gummy).
5. Stir or whisk in rosemary, salt, and pepper.

HONEY BARBECUE AIR FRIED SALMON

INGREDIENTS

Air Fried Salmon:

- 5 6oz. wild-caught skin-on salmon fillets
- 1 cup zero-sugar barbecue sauce
- 5 tsp. honey
- 1/2 tsp. paprika
- 1/2 tsp. cumin
- 1/2 tsp. onion powder

- 1/4 tsp sea salt
- Garlic Tomato Cauliflower Rice:
- 5 cups frozen cauliflower rice
- 1 1/2 tsp. minced garlic
- 3 tbsp diced white onion
- 1/2 cup cherry tomatoes
- 1 tsp. dried parsley

INSTRUCTIONS

1. Combine the honey and barbecue sauce in a small dish. In a separate small dish, whisk together the paprika, sea salt, cumin, & onion powder.
2. Pat the salmon fillets lightly with a paper towel & rub on the spice mixture to the side of the fillet without the skin.
3. Pour the honey barbecue mixture over the side of the salmon with the spice rub & spread evenly.
4. Air fry the salmon for 12 minutes at 360F.
5. For the Cauliflower Rice:
6. Heat a nonstick pan over medium heat. Drizzle with about 1 tbsp. olive oil.

7. Add in the minced garlic, white onion, and tomatoes. Cook for about 5 minutes or until the onions are slightly caramelized and translucent.
8. Add in the cauliflower rice and dried parsley.
9. Cover the pan and cook for another 5 minutes until the cauliflower rice is heated through and tender.

SWEET POTATO MISO SOUP

INGREDIENTS

- 1 piece Fresh Ginger ((about 2"))
- 3 med Sweet Potatoes
- 4 cups Vegetable Broth ((low sodium))
- 3 Tbs White Miso
- ½ cup Almond Milk ((unsweetened))
- ½ tsp Onion Powder
- ½ tsp Garlic Powder
- ½ tsp Salt

INSTRUCTIONS

1. Peel and mince the ginger
2. Saute ginger in a few tablespoons of veg broth until softened
3. Peel and boil the sweet potatoes for about 20 minutes or until soft
4. Drain the potatoes and mash
5. Add ginger,veggie broth, and spices and simmer for 10 minutes or so
6. Blend soup (immersion or blender) until smooth
7. Add miso to almond milk and whisk until smooth
8. Slowly stir in miso/milk mixture and heat for another minute or two
9. Add spices if necessary

BLUEBERRY PALEO MUFFINS

INGREDIENTS

- 2 cups blanched almond flour
- ½ cup coconut flour
- 1.5 teaspoons baking powder
- ½ cup fructose

- Pinch of salt
- 60g (2oz) dairy free butter
- 3 eggs
- ½ cup unsweetened almond milk
- 1 teaspoon vanilla bean extract
- 100g (3.5oz) blueberries

INSTRUCTIONS

1. Grease a 12 cup muffin pan or line the cups with paper baking cups
2. Preheat the oven to moderate (180°C/350°F)
3. Place the dairy free butter, vanilla bean extract and sugar in a bowl and mix well
4. Mix in the blanched almond flour, coconut flour, pinch of salt and baking powder
5. Add the eggs and almond milk, mixing well after each addition
6. Fold in the blueberries
7. Distribute the batter into the muffin cups and bake for about 30 minutes or until an inserted cake tester comes out clean.

HOMEMADE GRANOLA WITH CINNAMON & CARDAMON

INGREDIENTS

- 2 cup of jumbo oats
- 1/4 cup cashew butter or almond butter
- 1/4 cup maple syrup
- 1/4 cup coconut oil
- 4 tablespoons ground cinnamon
- 1 tablespoon ground cardamom
- 1 teaspoon vanilla
- 2 teaspoons sea salt
- 4 tablespoons pumpkin seeds
- 4 tablespoons flaked almonds
- Optional: 1/4 cup raisins or sultanas

INSTRUCTIONS

1. Preheat the oven to 170 C and line a baking tray with grease-proof paper.
2. Add the oats, seeds and nuts to a large bowl.
3. Melt the coconut oil in a frying pan over a low heat, then keep the heat on low and add the nut butter and maple syrup. Stir consistently until no lumps remain.

4. Remove the frying pan from the heat and stir in the cinnamon, cardamom, vanilla and sea salt.

5. Pour the wet mixture into the large bowl and mix until fully combined.

6. Spread the granola mixture into a very thin layer on the lined tray, using a spatula to press it together so that clumps form.

7. Bake for 25 minutes, then remove from the oven and stir to ensure even baking. Sprinkle over the raisins, and return to the oven for a further 10 minutes. Allow to cool fully before storing in an airtight container.

WILD PLANTAIN PANCAKES

INGREDIENTS

- 2 large green plantains or green bananas (or slightly yellow*)
- 2 large eggs
- 1 tablespoon coconut oil, plus more as needed (or grass-fed butter)
- Sea salt
- Grass-fed butter or coconut oil

INSTRUCTIONS

1. Run a knife up the plantain peel lengthwise, and pry your fingers between the plantain and peel to separate the peel away. Remove and discard peel.
2. Add 2 plantains and 2 eggs to the blender. Blend smooth, about 1 minute.
3. Melt a tablespoon of coconut oil in a skillet over medium heat. Add dollops of pancake batter to the skillet, and cook until the top starts to dry and the edges brown, about 2 - 4 minutes. Flip pancakes, and continue to cook until lightly browned with crisp edges.
4. If needed, add more coconut oil to the skillet between batches.
5. Top with grass-fed butter or coconut oil, and sprinkle with sea salt. Serve with a side of scrambled eggs, bacon, and a green smoothie.

ASIAN CHOPPED SALAD PEANUT GINGER DRESSING

INGREDIENTS

- Peanut Ginger Dressing
- 3 tablespoons ginger, peeled, chopped (or a 2-inch piece ginger root)
- ¼ cup rice wine vinegar
- 2 tablespoons canola oil
- 1 tablespoon soy sauce
- 1 tablespoons sesame oil
- 2 tablespoons peanut butter
- 1 teaspoon Siracha sauce
- ½ teaspoon orange zest
- 1/2 teaspoon ground coriander
- Asian Chopped Salad
- 3 cups red cabbage, chopped, about ½ head
- 3 green onions, sliced, use most of the onion
- 1 cup cucumber, ¼" dice
- 1 orange, peeled and diced (save some of the peel for zest in dressing)
- 1 cup carrot, shredded
- 1 cup edamame, steamed
- 1/4 cup chopped peanuts

INSTRUCTIONS

1. Combine all dressing ingredients in a blender or food processer and blend until smooth.
2. Assemble salad ingredients in a large bowl. Drizzle dressing over salad and toss to coat.

SKINNY LASAGNA SKILLET

INGREDIENTS

- 1 pound ground turkey
- 2 teaspoons olive oil
- salt and pepper to taste
- 1 teaspoon Italian seasoning
- ½ cup diced onion
- 1 ½ cups uncooked whole wheat pasta any short shape will work
- 2 cups marinara sauce
- 1 ½ cups water
- ½ cup shredded mozzarella cheese
- 1 tablespoon chopped parsley

INSTRUCTIONS

1. Heat the olive oil in a Dutch oven over medium-high heat. Add the onions and cook for 3 minutes. Add the ground turkey and season with salt and pepper to taste and the Italian seasoning.
2. Cook for 4-5 minutes until turkey is cooked through, using a spatula to break up the meat into bite-sized pieces.
3. Add the pasta, marinara sauce and water to the pan. Simmer for 11-12 minutes or until pasta is tender.
4. Preheat the broiler
5. Sprinkle the cheese over the top of the pasta and place under the broiler. Cook for 2-3 minutes or until cheese is melted. Top with parsley and serve.

HEALTHY LEMON CHICKEN AND SWEET POTATOES

INGREDIENTS

- 4 medium or 3 large sweet potatoes
- 3 chicken breasts boneless, skinless
- ½ cup fresh lemon juice (about 2 large lemons)
- ¼ cup olive oil
- 3 garlic cloves minced
- 1 tbsp Dijon mustard
- 1 tsp dried oregano
- 1 tsp turmeric
- ½ tsp salt
- ½ tsp black pepper
- 1 cup low-sodium chicken broth
- 1 large lemon sliced (optional)
- Parsley for garnish

INSTRUCTIONS

1. Preheat oven to 400 degrees F.
2. Cut sweet potatoes to desired size.* (see note)
3. In a mixing bowl, combine lemon juice, olive oil, minced garlic, Dijon mustard, oregano, turmeric, salt, black pepper, and chicken broth. Whisk to combine.
4. Arrange the sweet potatoes in a 9 x 13-inch baking pan. Place the chicken breasts over the sweet potatoes and pour lemon mixture on top. Top with lemon slices.
5. Roast in oven for 55-60 minutes. Top with chopped parsley and serve hot

BANANA CHOCOLATE CHIP SUNBUTTER COOKIES

INGREDIENTS

- 1/2 cup Sunbutter Or any nut butter of choice!
- 1 egg or 1/4 coconut oil (any oil of choice, except olive oil. It will make it rubbery and not a pleasant texture.)

- 1 banana more brown = sweeter the taste
- 1 tbsp pure maple syrup or coconut sugar (OPTIONAL) For a little sweeter taste.
- 1/4 cup flour I used Bob's Red Mill GF Cup for Cup Flour, feel free to use ANY flour to make it grain free. It is just to thicken up the sunbutter.
- 1/2 tsp baking soda
- 1/4 tsp salt OMIT if you have a salty nut butter.
- 1/4 cup chocolate chips I prefer Enjoy Life Dark Chocolate Morsels, any sugar free dark chocolate is a great contrast to the sweet banana.

INSTRUCTIONS

1. Preheat oven to 350 Degrees Fahrenheit
2. Line baking sheet with wax paper or something to prevent it from sticking. (I use a reusable silicone mat.)
3. Mash banana, egg, and and Sunbutter together.
4. Stir flour, and baking soda together.

5. Combine dry ingredients with wet ingredients. See my video below for the next couple steps.

6. (Learn from my mistakes! Do it separately first!)

7. Fold in chocolate chips. (I do this last in order to minimize chunks of flour in the previous mixing process.)

8. Bake for 10 minutes.

9. (If you don't believe in preheating, probably 12 minutes. But try to believe in preheating!)

10. It will naturally look golden brown, so look for how firm the cookie looks. Take them a little underbaked for that soft and gooey center.

11. Allow to cool for a minute, if you can stand it. I always pop one in my mouth the second it isn't scorching hot. (If it cools too much you can microwave it for 5-8 seconds to warm it up.)

GREEK TURKEY BURGERS WITH TZATZIKI SAUCE

INGREDIENTS

For the Turkey Burgers:

- 1 pound ground turkey
- ½ cup fresh spinach leaves , chopped
- ⅓ cup sun-dried tomatoes , chopped
- 1/4 cup red onion , minced
- ¼ cup feta cheese , crumbled
- 2 cloves garlic , pressed or minced
- 1 egg , whisked
- 1 tablespoon olive oil
- 1 teaspoon dried oregano
- 1/2 teaspoon kosher salt
- 1/2 teaspoon freshly ground black pepper
- 4 soft whole-wheat hamburger buns
- Bibb lettuce leaves
- Sliced red onion
- For the Tzatziki Sauce:

INSTRUCTIONS

1. In a large bowl, add the ground turkey, spinach, sun-dried tomatoes, red onion and feta. In a small bowl, whisk together the garlic, egg, olive oil and dried oregano and kosher salt and freshly ground black pepper then pour over the turkey and mix with your hands to combine.

2. Divide the burger mixture into 4 portions and mold into patties. Place on a cutting board or plate dividing the patties with parchment paper and refrigerated for 30 minutes up to overnight. You could also individually freeze the patties at this point for up to 3 months.

3. Prepare the tzatziki sauce by grating the cucumber. Gather the cucumber together and place in a paper towel and press the water out of the shredded cucumber and place in a medium size bowl. Add the yogurt, garlic, red wine vinegar, fresh dill, kosher salt and freshly ground black pepper and mix well. Cover and refrigerate for 30 minutes or up to 3 days.

4. Heat a non-stick grill pan over medium heat and spray well with cooking spray.

5. Place the turkey burgers on the grill, cover with an upside down sheet pan or lid and cook for about 5 minutes per side. Be sure to watch the burgers and monitor your heat as the burgers will brown quickly if the heat is too high.

6. Slather buns with tzatziki sauce and garnish with lettuce leaves and red onion. Or serve bunless in the bibb lettuce leaves.

CILANTRO-LIME HONEY GARLIC SHRIMP

INGREDIENTS

- 1 tablespoon olive oil
- 1 tablespoon butter
- 1 lb shrimp (20-25 count, uncooked, deveined, peeled, tails-on)
- 3 garlic cloves , minced
- 4 tablespoons honey
- 3 tablespoons lime juice freshly squeezed
- 1 tablespoon soy sauce
- 3 tablespoons cilantro chopped

INSTRUCTIONS

1. In a large skillet, heat olive oil and butter. Add shrimp and minced garlic and cook for 5 minutes, occasionally turning shrimp over, until shrimp is cooked.
2. In a small bowl, combine honey, lime juice, soy sauce, and chopped cilantro. Mix to combine.
3. Add the mixture to the skillet with shrimp. Bring to high heat, coat the shrimp with the mixture, and cook for about 1-2 minutes until the sauce reduces just a touch. Remove from heat. Let it stand for sauce to thicken.

ORANGE BROWN BUTTER SHRIMP

INGREDIENTS

- 1/2 cup butter
- 1 teaspoon fresh thyme
- zest of one orange
- 2 teaspoons minced garlic
- 2 lbs. raw shrimp
- 1/2 teaspoon chili powder
- salt and pepper to taste

INSTRUCTIONS

1. Heat the butter in a medium skillet over low heat. When the butter is melted, add the thyme leaves. Stir and simmer, keeping the heat low (it burns easily), for 5 minutes or until the butter reaches a golden brown color. Remove from heat and stir in the zest. Pour the butter into a small bowl and let it rest for a few minutes.

2. In the same skillet, with a light coating of the butter remaining, add the garlic and saute for 1 minute. Add the raw shrimp and the chili powder; shake or toss in the pan for 3-5 minutes or until the shrimp is no longer translucent. Serve with the butter and pasta, grains, rice, or a salad.

ONE POT LEMON ORZO WITH SHRIMP

INGREDIENTS

- 1 lb raw shrimp, peeled and deveined
- kosher salt and freshly ground black pepper to taste
- olive oil

- 1 medium onion, diced
- 3 cloves garlic, minced
- 1 tsp dried basil
- 1/2 tsp dried oregano
- 8 oz dried orzo pasta
- 2 1/4 cups regular chicken broth
- 1 (14.5 oz) can diced tomatoes, juices reserved (approx 1/4 cup)
- 1/2 cup broccoli florets, bite size
- juice of 1 medium lemon
- 1/4 cup freshly shaved/grated parmesan cheese

INSTRUCTIONS

1. Towel dry the shrimp. Sprinkle with a pinch of kosher salt and freshly ground black pepper, toss, and set aside.
2. In a large oven-proof pan, heat 2 TB olive oil over medium high heat. Add onion, garlic, basil, oregano, and stir about 3 minutes. Stir in orzo and continue stirring about 1 minute.
3. Stir in chicken broth and 1/4 cup reserved tomato juice. Bring to a boil, cover, and

reduce to simmer. Simmer just until pasta is under al dente, about 7 minutes. Stir in tomatoes, broccoli, and lemon juice. Stir in shrimp. Cover and simmer for 5 minutes. Stir again and simmer 1 minute longer if needed, just until shrimp turns opaque.

4. Serve immediately with fresh parmesan.

CHOCOLATE CHIP GREEK YOGURT PANCAKES

INGREDIENTS

- 2 cups white whole wheat flour
- 2 teaspoons baking powder
- 1/2 teaspoon baking soda
- 1/2 teaspoon salt
- 1 cup vanilla Greek yogurt
- 1 cup milk
- 2 large eggs
- 2 tablespoons oil
- 3 tablespoons honey
- 1 teaspoon vanilla extract
- 1/2 cup mini chocolate chips

INSTRUCTIONS

1. Heat a large skillet or griddle to medium heat and spray well with non stick cooking spray.
2. In a large bowl, mix together the flour, baking powder, baking soda, and salt.
3. In a separate bowl, mix together the greek yogurt, milk, eggs, oil, honey, and vanilla.
4. Add the dry ingredients to the wet ingredients and mix until just combined, making sure not to over mix the batter. Gently fold in the chocolate chips.
5. Using a ¼ cup measuring cup, scoop the batter from the bowl and drop onto the skillet or griddle. Once the top starts to bubble and the edges look set, flip and let cook for another 1-2 minutes.
6. Serve with extra chocolate chips, fresh fruit, or pure maple syrup!

PEANUT BUTTER AND HONEY BANANA MUFFINS

INGREDIENTS

- 2 large ripe bananas
- 3/4 cup peanut butter I prefer chunky, but smooth is also fine
- 1/2 cup Plain Greek Yogurt
- 1/4 cup honey
- 1/4 cup maple syrup
- 1/4 cup almond or flax milk coconut, rice, hemp, or soy is also fine
- 1 large egg
- 2 tsp vanilla extract
- 1 3/4 cup all purpose flour or whole wheat flour
- 2 tsp cinnamon
- 1 tsp baking powder
- 1 tsp baking soda
- 1/4 tsp salt
- 1/4 cup chia seeds optional

INSTRUCTIONS

1. Preheat oven to 375 degrees. Line a 12 cup muffin tin with muffin liners, or generously grease a muffin tin with cooking spray.
2. With a fork or pastry knife, mash up your bananas (no chunks) and place in a large bowl. Add peanut butter, honey, maple syrup, yogurt, milk, egg, and vanilla extract. Beat with an electric mixture until smooth. Set aside.
3. In a medium bowl, mix together the remaining (dry) ingredients. Add the dry ingredients to the wet, and mix with a rubber spatular until well combined and the flour pockets have disappeared.
4. Fill muffin cups to about 3/4 full (or more if you have leftover batter).
5. Bake for 15-18 minutes or until the tops are golden brown and a toothpick inserted in the middle comes out clean. Mine take right around 16 minutes!

COCONUT CURRY CHICKEN (SLOW COOKER)

INGREDIENTS

Crockpot Curry Chicken

- 1.5 lbs. boneless, skinless chicken breast
- 1 tablespoon minced garlic
- 1 15-oz. can full-fat coconut milk
- 3 tablespoons green curry paste
- 1/2 teaspoon garlic powder
- 1/8 teaspoon salt (or more, to taste)
- 1/2 teaspoon chili powder
- 2 tablespoons fresh Thai basil or cilantro
- 2 tablespoons fresh lime juice, or more to taste
- Peppers and Onions
- 1 large green pepper, sliced
- 1 large red pepper, sliced
- 1/2 medium red onion, sliced
- 1 tablespoon coconut oil
- 1/8 teaspoon salt
- 1/8 teaspoon ground pepper

INSTRUCTIONS

1. Place the minced garlic, coconut milk, curry paste, garlic powder, salt, and chili powder into the slow cooker and whisk everything together until combined.
2. Submerge the chicken breast in the sauce, making sure that both sides get coated.
3. Cover the slow cooker and cook on low for 6-8 hours (recommended), high for 2-4 hours
4. When there are about 20 minutes left of cook time for the chicken, prepare the peppers and onions.
5. Heat coconut oil in a large skillet over medium/high heat.
6. Then, add the sliced veggies and sauté for about 5 minutes, just enough to flash fry them so they aren't soggy. Season with salt and pepper. Remove from heat.
7. Once the chicken has cooked all the way through and has an internal temperature of 165°F, remove and shred chicken with 2 forks.

8. Place the shredded chicken back into slow cooker with the sauce and mix. Add the cooked peppers and onions and fresh lime juice to the slow cooker and toss everything together.

9. Serve with Thai basil or cilantro with your favorite grain.

ITALIAN LEMON ALMOND FLOUR CAKE (TORTA CAPRESE BIANCA - GRAIN-FREE, GLUTEN-FREE)

INGREDIENTS

- 320 grams (this is about 3 cups + 3 tablespoons) almond flour (not almond meal) or blanched almonds, ground into almond flour
- 200 grams (1 cup + 3 tablespoons) white chocolate, chopped
- 2 tablespoons whipping cream or milk (I used 1.5% milk)
- 180 grams (3/4 cup + 1 tablespoon) unsalted butter, softened
- 130 grams (about 2/3 cup) granulated sugar or coconut sugar1, divided

- zest of 4 lemons, about 2 tablespoons
- 4 large eggs, separated
- 1 teaspoon lemon extract
- 40 grams (about 2 tablespoons) of limoncello or lemon juice
- berries and powdered sugar as garnish, optional

INSTRUCTIONS

1. Preheat your oven to 350°F / 176°C and grease a 10" / 26cm pan or line it with parchment paper. If using blanched almonds instead of almond flour, process them in the food processor until they're pretty finely ground. If you grind them too much, they'll release oil and become almond butter.
2. Combine the white chocolate and milk / cream in a microwave safe bowl.
3. Heat in 30 second increments and stir after every 30 seconds. Set aside to cool while you prepare the rest. Beat the butter with 100 grams of sugar and beat until fluffy.
4. Add the lemon zest, egg yolks and lemon extract and beat until well combined. Then

add the almond flour / ground almonds and the melted chocolate. Add the limoncello / lemon juice and beat until combined.

5. In a separate bowl with spotlessly clean beaters, beat the egg whites until soft peaks form. Gradually add the remaining 30 grams of sugar to the egg white mixture. Fold the egg whites into the almond batter until well combined. Spoon the batter into the greased pan and bake for 40 - 45 minutes. If making half the cake, use a 7" / 18cm pan and bake for 30 minutes. The cake will puff up in the oven, but when cooling, it'll fall back down.

6. Let it cool completely in the pan and then invert the cake onto a plate, and then flip that back into the pan or onto another plate (so that it's not upside down). Sprinkle on some powdered sugar if desired and top with berries, but only before serving. Cake can be stored at room temperature for up to 3 days or refrigerated (I think it's best that way) for up to 5.

3-INGREDIENT COCONUT OIL BISCUITS

INGREDIENTS

- 2 cups self-rising flour, store-bought or homemade
- 1/4 cup coconut oil (solid, not melted)
- 3/4 cup milk*

INSTRUCTIONS

1. Preheat oven to 425 degrees.
2. Add self-rising flour and coconut oil to a mixing bowl, and use a pastry cutter or forks to cut the coconut oil into the flour until the mixture is like fine crumbs. Stir in the milk until mixture forms a soft dough and no longer sticks to the sides of the bowl. Knead the mixture until combined, but be careful not to over-knead.
3. Turn the dough out onto a cutting board that has been lightly dusted with flour. Gently roll the dough out until it reaches a 1/2-inch thickness. Use a biscuit cutter (mine was a 2-inch circle) to cut out the biscuits, and transfer to a baking sheet.

4. Bake for 10 minutes, or until the biscuits have risen and ever so slightly begin to brown on top. Remove and serve immediately.

CHICKEN TETRAZINI

INGREDIENTS

- 1 12 ounce box pasta
- 2 cooked and chopped chicken breasts
- 3 T butter
- ½ C shredded zucchini (optional)
- ½ C shredded carrots (optional)
- ¼ cup minced onion (optional)
- 2 T minced garlic
- 1 can (fat free) cream of chicken soup
- ½ C reduced fat sour cream
- ½ C skim milk
- ½ C reduced fat Parmesan cheese
- salt and pepper to taste
- dry parsley to garnish (optional)

INSTRUCTIONS

1. While the pasta is boiling, melt butter on low heat in a frying pan.
2. Add garlic, onion, zucchini, and carrots. Saute for about 3 minutes.
3. Add soup, sour cream, milk, cheese, and chicken. Stir over low heat until pasta is done boiling. Drain pasta and add to the mixture. Toss well and serve immediately.

CHOCOLATE CHIP BANANA OAT MUFFINS (VEGAN, GLUTEN FREE).

INGREDIENTS

- 1 cup gluten free flour
- ¾ cup oat flour
- ½ teaspoon baking soda
- ¾ teaspoon baking powder
- ½ teaspoon salt
- ¾ cup organic cane sugar or coconut sugar
- ⅓ cup melted vegan buttery spread or coconut oil
- 2 ripe bananas mashed (about ¾ cups)
- 1 teaspoon vanilla extract

- 1 teaspoon apple cider vinegar
- ¼ cup water
- ¾ cup dairy free mini chocolate chips I used the Enjoy Life brand

INSTRUCTIONS

1. Preheat the oven to 350 degrees. Line a muffin pan with paper cupcake liners.
2. Place the bananas in a bowl, and mash them thoroughly. Add the sugar and stir. Add the melted vegan buttery spread, water, vanilla extract, and vinegar. Stir to combine.
3. Add the gluten free flour, oat flour, baking powder, baking soda, and salt. Stir well.
4. Add the chocolate chips to the bowl and stir gently.
5. Spoon the batter into the prepared muffin pan, filling each cup about ⅔ full.
6. Bake at 350 degrees for 20-23 minutes, until the tops are golden brown. You can insert a toothpick in the middle of a muffin to make sure that it's done - it should come out clean.
7. Allow to cool in the pan for at least 15 minutes before removing.

GRILLED PESTO POTATOES

INGREDIENTS

To make the basil pesto:

- 2 cups fresh basil leaves packed
- 1/2 cup freshly grated Parmesan-Reggiano cheese
- 1/2 cup extra virgin olive oil
- 1/4 cup pine nuts
- 2 garlic cloves minced
- Salt and freshly ground black pepper to taste

For the Potatoes:

- 5 red potatoes washed and cut into cubes
- Cooking Spray
- Aluminum Foil

INSTRUCTIONS

1. Combine the basil, garlic, and pine nuts in a food processor or blender and pulse until coarsely chopped. With the machine running, slowly add the olive oil and process until smooth. Add the cheese and pulse until

combined. Season with salt and pepper, to taste.

2. In a medium bowl, combine potatoes and pesto. Mix until potatoes are well covered. Spray a large piece of aluminum foil with cooking spray. Add the potatoes and wrap in a foil packet. Wrap another piece of foil around the packet so it is sturdy enough to grill.

3. Preheat the grill to medium-high heat. Place the potato packet on the grill. Cook for 15 minutes and then flip the packet. Cook for an additional 15 minutes, or until potatoes are tender and slightly crisp. Carefully remove the potatoes from the packet and serve warm.

GLAZED PUMPKIN SPICE SCONES

INGREDIENTS

- 1 3/4 cups flour
- 1/3 cup sugar
- 2 tsp baking powder
- 1/2 tsp baking soda
- 1/4 tsp salt

- 1 tsp cinnamon
- 1/8 tsp cloves
- 1/8 tsp ginger
- 1/8 tsp nutmeg
- 1/4 cup chilled unsalted butter
- 1/2 cup pure pumpkin
- 2 Tbsp low-fat buttermilk
- 1 large egg
- 1/2 tsp vanilla extract
- Glaze
- 1 cup powdered sugar, sifted
- 1/4 tsp cinnamon
- 1 1/2 Tbsp milk
- 1 Tbsp unsalted butter, melted
- 1 Tbsp vanilla extract

INSTRUCTIONS

1. Preheat oven to 400°F and line a baking sheet with a silicone mat or parchment paper. Whisk together flour, sugar, baking powder, baking soda, salt, and spices in a large bowl. Dice butter into 1/2-inch pieces; sprinkle over flour mixture and use a pastry

cutter to cut in evenly until mixture resembles coarse meal.

2. Whisk together pumpkin, buttermilk, egg, and vanilla in a small bowl; add to flour mixture and fold in just until incorporated. Use a floured bench scraper to scrape dough out onto prepared baking sheet; flour hands and pat dough into an 8-inch circle. Score into 12 wedges with floured bench scraper.

3. Bake 16 to 17 minutes, until golden. Cool 2 minutes on baking sheet, then carefully transfer to wire rack to cool before slicing into wedges. To prepare glaze, combine powdered sugar, cinnamon, milk, butter, and vanilla in a small bowl. Set rack with scones over a piece of wax paper and drizzle with glaze; let set before serving. If not serving scones immediately, store unglazed in an airtight container up to 2 days and glaze just before serving.

EASY BANANA PUDDING

INGREDIENTS

- 2 medium bananas (peeled)
- 1 tsp. honey (optional)
- ½ tsp. pure vanilla extract (optional)
- 1 tbsp. walnuts (optional - for topping)

INSTRUCTIONS

1. Blend the bananas until they become like pudding. I find using a stick blender to be easiest, but you can pulse this in a regular blender or food processor as well.
2. Mix in any optional additions and serve with optional toppings Get creative!

BLUEBERRY THUMBPRINT COOKIES

INGREDIENTS

- Filling:
- 2 cups blueberries
- 1 Tbsp Maple Syrup
- ¼ cup Water
- ¼ cup Lemon Juice
- ½ tsp Nutmeg
- 1 tsp Cinnamon
- 1-2 Tbsp Arrowroot Powder
- Cookie:
- 2 cup Blanched Almond Flour
- 1 cup Arrowroot Powder, plus ½ cup for dusting
- 1 tsp Salt
- 1 tsp Pure Vanilla Extract
- ⅓ cup Maple Syrup
- ¼ cup Organic Coconut Oil, melted

INSTRUCTIONS

1. In a medium sized sauce pan, add the blueberries, syrup, water, lemon juice,

nutmeg and cinnamon. Heat over medium heat.

2. Bring filling to a boil, while stirring. Continue to stir frequently, while "mashing" the filling with a wooded spoon.

3. Once the liquid has reduced, turn heat down and add arrowroot powder. Stir continuously until thickned. Remove from heat and set aside for filling the cookies. Can add additional ½ cup blueberries if desired.

4. Preheat oven to 350 degrees.

5. In a large mixing bowl, stir together the almond flour, arrowroot, and salt.

6. Add in the vanilla extract, maple syrup, and melted coconut oil. Stir until all ingredients are combined and you have a ball of cookie dough.

7. Prepare a baking sheet lined with parchment paper.

8. Take a small ball of dough and roll until about the size of a ping-pong ball. Use extra arrow root powder when working with the dough if necessary.

9. Place on cookie sheet and press thumb into center making a well.

10. Add about a teaspoon (give or take) of filling to the center of the cookies.

11. Repeat until all dough has been used.

12. Place in the oven and bake cookies for 20 minutes.

13. Remove from oven and place on a cooling rack.

14. Any remaining filling can be refrigerated or frozen and saved for future use.

CHICKEN AND AVOCADO SALAD WITH LIME AND CILANTRO

INGREDIENTS

- 3 cups cooked chicken, cut into large pieces
- 2 medium avocados, diced
- 3 T fresh squeezed lime juice, divided
- salt, to taste
- 1/4 cup thinly sliced green onion
- 1/2 cup finely chopped fresh cilantro (see notes)
- 3 T mayo (see notes)

INSTRUCTIONS

1. Cut up enough chicken to make 3 cups of chopped chicken. I like it cut into fairly large chunks.
2. Dice the avocados into medium-sized pieces, put in small bowl, mix with 1 T of the lime juice, and season avocado with salt to taste.
3. Thinly slice the green onion and finely chop the cilantro (if using).
4. Mix 3 T mayo and 2 T lime juice to make the dressing. (If you're not a huge lime fan like I am, you might want to start with less lime and taste, adding more until it seems sour enough for you.
5. Put the chicken into a bowl large enough to hold all the salad ingredients.
6. Add the sliced green onions and dressing and toss until all the chicken is coated with dressing.
7. Add the avocado and any lime juice in the bottom of the bowl and gently combine with the chicken.

8. Then add the chopped cilantro and gently mix into the salad, just until it is barely combined. Season with salt to taste.

9. Serve right away or chill for a while before serving. This could be served inside pita bread or sandwich bread, or inside crisp lettuce cups, but we just ate it as a salad.

10. This will keep in the fridge overnight, but the avocado is best when it's freshly made. When I make it I rarely have leftovers, but if you're only making for one or two people you might want to cut the recipe in half.

HONEY GLAZED CARROTS

INGREDIENTS

- 1 lb baby carrots
- 2 Tbsp high heat oil see above for why I like to use avocado oil
- 2 Tbsp honey
- 1 Tbsp lemon juice
- black pepper to taste
- 1 Tbsp parsley

INSTRUCTIONS

1. In a medium saucepan, bring water to a boil.
2. Add the carrots and cook until they are tender, about 5-6 minutes.
3. Drain the water from saucepan and return it to stove.
4. Add oil, honey, and lemon juice to the pot and turn your stove's temperature to medium heat. (If you have a stove with numbered dials 1-9, I would pick a 5).
5. Cook until the glaze coats the carrots, usually about 5 minutes.
6. Season with pepper and garnish with parsley for color and an extra nutrient punch.

MY SUPER EASY GLUTEN-FREE PAD THAI RECIPE (GUT-FRIENDLY AND DAIRY-FREE TOO)

INGREDIENTS

- 2 cups of rice noodles (pre-cooked or dry depending on preference)
- 2 chicken breasts, diced
- 1 courgette

- 1 tablespoon of coconut oil, or olive oil if preferred
- 1-2 tablespoons of chicken seasoning
- 2 tablespoons of gluten-free soy sauce.
- 1 thumbsize piece of ginger.
- 1 garlic clove.
- 1-2 slices of lime
- 1 teaspoon of cashew nut butter
- Nutritonal Yeast, optional
- 1 teaspoon of turmeric, optional
- Black pepper for seasoning, optional

INSTRUCTIONS

1. Add 2 tablespoons of coconut oil to frying pan and heat.
2. Finely chop ginger and garlic and add to pan. Cook until they brown.
3. Peel and finely slice courgette and add this to the pan.
4. Add diced chicken, and chicken seasoning. cook until lightly browned (around 6-8 minutes)
5. Add in noodles (if you buy dry rice noodles; you'll need to boil these in water beforehand

for five minutes) and stir fry with chicken and courgette for 2 minutes.

6. Add soy sauce, turmeric and squeeze over the juice of 1 slice of lime.

7. Add 1 teaspoon of nut butter and melt in pan, stirring through.

8. Turn pan off heat. Add in a sprinkle of black pepper, nutritional yeast and a final squeeze of lime.

BANANA CUPCAKES

INGREDIENTS

FOR THE BANANA CUPCAKES

- 1 ¼ cups very ripe bananas mashed
- 1 pkg white cake mix
- 2 eggs
- 1 teaspoon baking soda
- 2/3 cup water
- 1 tablespoon vinegar
- 2/3 cup walnuts optional

FOR THE CREAM CHEESE FROSTING

- 2 tablespoons cream cheese
- milk
- 4 cups powdered sugar
- 4 tablespoons butter softened
- 1 teaspoon vanilla extract

INSTRUCTIONS

To Make the Banana Cupcakes

1. Preheat your oven to 350 degrees.
2. Mix together water, vinegar and baking soda. Combine with cake mix and eggs. Stir until well combined, and scrape the bowl with spatula.
3. Add the mashed bananas. Mix all with an electric mixer for 3 minutes at medium speed.
4. Pour into lined cupcake pan. Bake at 350 degrees for 35 minutes or until a toothpick comes out clean.
5. When cooled, frost with the Cream Cheese Frosting.

BROILED TILAPIA WITH PARMESAN

INGREDIENTS

- 4 Tilapia Fillets (defrosted if frozen)
- 1/4 Cup Parmesan Cheese
- 1/4 Cup Plain Non-Fat or Low-Fat Greek Yogurt
- 1 Tablespoon Fresh Lemon Juice
- 1/2 Teaspoon Fresh Dill
- Pepper to taste

INSTRUCTIONS

1. Turn your oven's broiler onto high and adjust oven rack to the top.
2. In a small bowl, combine all ingredients except the tilapia. Set aside.
3. Place tilapia fillets on a baking sheet lined with aluminum foil or parchment paper to avoid sticking.
4. Broil the fish on one side for three minutes.
5. Remove the pan from the oven, flip fish over and divide the parmesan mixture over the uncooked sides of the tilapia.

6. Return fish to the oven and broil an additional 3-4 minutes making sure not to over cook the fish.

EVERYDAY ZUCCHINI

INGREDIENTS

- zucchini
- olive oil
- italian seasoning
- salt and pepper

INSTRUCTIONS

1. Rinse enough vegetables for however many people you are serving, 1 medium zucchini for every two people.
2. Quarter the zucchini lengthwise and then chop into half inch sections. Film enough olive oil in a large sauté pan to just barely film the bottom.
3. No more than a few tablespoons, depending on how much zucchini you have.

4. Set the pan over a strong medium to medium high heat.
5. Sprinkle with salt, pepper, and a generous amount of italian seasoning. Again, judge this on preference and the amount you are cooking. Leave the veggies where they are for several minutes to acquire some color on them.
6. If they are just kind of steaming, turn up the heat a bit. Give them a toss, and then leave them alone again to get more color on a different side.
7. Pull them from the heat when they are fairly well browned but have not become mushy.
8. Taste for salt and pepper and serve immediately.

LOADED BRUSSEL SPROUT SALAD (GLUTEN FREE, DAIRY FREE)

INGREDIENTS

For the Salad:

- 1 cup quinoa
- 1–2 chicken breasts, seasonings to taste

- 3 pieces bacon
- About 20 brussel sprouts
- handful of asparagus
- 2 bunches of kale
- 1 tbsp garlic
- 1/4 red onion
- Feta cheese (optional)
- For the Dressing:
- 1/2 cup olive oil
- 1 tbsp dijon mustard
- 1/4 cup lemon juice

INSTRUCTIONS

1. Cook quinoa. Add 1 cup of quinoa + 2 cups of water, boil on medium-high for about 10 minutes, until all the water is absorbed into quinoa.
2. Prepare chicken in any way you choose, such as pan frying with salt and pepper. I used shredded chicken I had made for a different recipe in the crockpot.
3. Preheat oven to 410 degrees and place strips of bacon on baking sheet and cook for 15 minutes or until crispy. You can also use

bacon bits or bacon you have previously made.

4. While the bacon and quinoa cook, thinly slice brussel sprouts, chop asparagus, and shred kale. Combine in a large bowl and toss in olive oil, garlic, salt and pepper.

5. Remove bacon. Place the brussel sprouts, asparagus, and kale on baking sheet and bake for roughly 20 minutes.

6. While these bake, chop the bacon and thinly slice the red onion.

7. Combine the quinoa, chicken, red onion, bacon, asparagus, kale and brussel sprouts.

8. Pour dressing over the salad, add feta (if using), and toss!

9. Refrigerate for a few hours (up to 24 hours, but you may need to add more dressing).

LOW FODMAP GRANOLA MUESLI

INGREDIENTS

- 2 and ½ cups (200g) rolled oats (gluten free)
- 1 cup (30g) corn flakes (gluten free)
- 1 cup (30g) plain rice puffs (gluten free)
- ¼ cup (30g) sliced or slivered almonds
- ¼ cup (30g) roughly chopped pecan nuts
- ¼ cup (40g) roughly chopped hazelnuts
- ¼ cup (35g) sunflower seeds
- ¼ cup (35g) pumpkin seeds (pepitas)
- 2 tablespoons chia seeds
- ½ teaspoon cinnamon
- 1 teaspoon vanilla bean paste (alternative 1 tablespoon pure vanilla essence)
- ⅓ cup (80 ml) coconut oil, liquid form
- ½ cup (125 ml) pure maple syrup

INSTRUCTIONS

1. Preheat the oven at 160° (320 F°)
2. In a bowl mix together all dry ingredients
3. Stir in the maple syrup, vanilla bean paste and the coconut oil
4. Spread the mixture thinly and evenly on a baking tray covered by baking paper
5. Bake in the oven for about 45 minutes, stirring every 15 minutes or so
6. Remove from oven when it has a golden colour and it's crispy in texture
7. Break up any big chunks
8. Cool down, use what you need and store the remaining in an airtight container for up to 10 days
9. Serve with your favourite low FODMAP milk